Crazy Rich Health

No Fads, No Diets
Easy
At Any Age

Charles Harwood

Publisher's Note:

This book is not designed to be a substitute for medical advice. The reader should consult their physician or nurse practitioner in matters relating to their health, particularly with respect to any symptoms that may require diagnosis.

Contents

Preface

I'm grateful for so many things every day but one of the biggest might be that I have chosen to realize that no one is responsible for my health and happiness but me. Certainly, I can't know about all the myriad of possible life scenarios faced by people around the world, but I do know that, for most, there is much to be gained by not giving your health, your happiness or your life up to anyone or anything.

Once we give up the responsibility for our health to our doctor, our next prescription, the government or even our genetics then we start giving up our chance for *Crazy Rich Health*. The default setting for our body is healthy.

Default – a preselected option adopted by a mechanism when no alternative is specified by the user or programmer.

I have certainly known bad health, obesity and being a hypochondriac and I believe I experienced all the excuses possible for not turning my life around. Fortunately, I finally realized that we are all the programmers of our bodies and unless we change the settings by our actions, we will enjoy that good health. **But what can change those settings?** After years, I figured out all the ways I had changed my settings and I'll tell you what I learned because I really want you to know. I came to realize that so much of happiness was what I chose to think about and focus upon. Although I might not have liked something someone said or did, it was up to me how I felt about it. It's the same with health in that it's about our choices and what we focus on as important when it comes to how our body feels. **But what are good choices and what are unhealthy ones?** I will tell you that because I really want you to know that as well.

> Speaking of desire and MONEY, Jeff Bezos, the founder of Amazon, had a desire to do something big. He said, 'I don't want to be 80 years old and in a quiet moment of reflection, thinking back over my life and cataloging a bunch of major regrets.' He is now worth more at $140 billion than the $82 billion book market he set out to disrupt. Desire, focused desire. No regret!

Money is no different from good health in that most of us equate good health with one of its attributes like more energy, better looks, no sickness, slowed aging, ideal weight or protection from those diseases that may show up later in life such a heart disease, cancer, Alzheimer's and diabetes.

What is your Why? Do you know?

And please be willing to remain open to ideas you may not have considered before. Let me repeat that because it's very important. **You need to be open to ideas you may not have considered before.**

For the best results you'll need to be honest with yourself. Like I said earlier, even if you're looking for an excuse to continue a life that you really know is not your best, maybe I can help to change that. Certainly, if you know you want to eliminate the roadblocks that may have been holding you back—Let's Do This! The possibilities are amazing.

First - Know that Rationalization is not your friend!

Rationalize: to attempt to explain or justify (one's own or another's behavior or attitude) with logical, plausible reasons, even if these are not true or appropriate.

Boy, can I tell you about rationalization! And about many people's two best friends - in their mission to do what they want without admitting it's not their best choice - sugar and alcohol (sugar). Well, there is cannabis and... You get the idea.

> Speaking of marijuana – I'm not necessarily advocating it, but did you know that marijuana has 34 elements that are beneficial in the treatment of cancer and it is NOT FDA approved?
>
> Chemotherapy was discovered by attempting to poison people with mustard gas and IS FDA approved.
>
> I'm not denying that discoveries (like chemotherapy) can't be made through strange avenues, but I do wonder why chemotherapy with potentially challenging side effects and varied success rates has been approved and a natural plant with virtually no side effects was not? Fortunately for many, medical marijuana is now available, as of this writing, in 33 states, while 10 states and Washington, DC have legalized it for recreational use.

Check the appendix - for a bonus on Desire

Second - Denial can be a tool or a crutch!

Denial ain't just a river in Egypt –

- Mark Twain

Denial can be a useful tool in times of extreme grief or stress, but at some point we have got to be honest with ourselves. We can't expect our lives to change if we don't. I do believe that sometimes denial is not wanting to accept a limitation that others might want to place on you, and that might be a good thing. Just because someone else says so doesn't make them right.

Third - Belief is what makes you who you are.

*If you don't change your beliefs, your life will
be like this forever. Is that good news?*

- W. Somerset Maugham

If you're interested in making changes in your life, you may have to change some of your beliefs. Our beliefs come mainly from our experiences and our education and many of us may have found beliefs we needed to change. There are beliefs of fact and beliefs of faith and, remember, both are subject to change. A fact, in some cases, is only a fact because that's the general consensus. So when most of the people around you believe something it can be hard to make changes. When you are ready to move away from what everybody else believes, consider this:

*Until Roger Banister ran the mile in under four minutes
(3:59.4) it was said by many "experts" that it was not
possible.*

Although there's no real evidence that Einstein really said it, as many believe, I still love this expression **Insanity is doing the same thing over and over and expecting different results.** That's something else I know about too and I guess, for me, it was not knowing, or not trying hard enough to know, what to do differently. At that time, my good friends denial, procrastination, rationalization and Gallo burgundy wine were very helpful with keeping myself insane. Fortunately, enough profound events snapped me out of it.

I really love talking about belief. The word belief comes from two words. 'Be' comes from being and 'lief' from leubh, which means love. So belief really means to be in love with. You may not need to know whether something you believe is a fact, but you do need to love it. Very powerful stuff!

Check the appendix for a bonus on belief.

Fourth – Focus is the magic tool that keeps it all together and helps us to move forward.

Follow One Course Until Successful

I would have to say if anything has been an obsession for me most of my life, it would be learning to be focused. Not just in the context of staying the singular course but in so many ways. As I have gotten better and better at being focused in the here and now, it has opened up new worlds that I want to share with you. More on that later and check out the appendix for a bonus on focus.

My ultimate goal is to show you that *Crazy Rich Health* can be so much easier to achieve than you think. I had to learn to be healthy but I did and now I have a great life—mainly because I am very healthy, which has the side benefit of my being very happy. My health does not come from following some ancient restrictive diet or having great wealth, instead it comes from understanding the value of keeping it simple.

In 1776 when Benjamin Franklin said, 'An ounce of prevention is worth a pound of cure,' he was actually warning Philadelphia about fire safety. Today we use it more to make a point about staying healthy. I'm sure you would like to hold on to good health rather than trying to get it back. But that being said, I also believe

It ain't over till it's over, if you know how to get it back!

I am so excited for you and I really hope you'll allow what I have to say to improve your life in amazing ways. Don't let your health fall to the wayside because you ignored the messages from your body and didn't cherish the gift of wellbeing. Don't regret not giving your life what it needs to be Great!

Here we go. And of course, the FDA has not approved this message. And if you have any doubts about any ideas or suggestions that follow, feel free to check with your doctor AND do your own research. Or perhaps check with your results.

Oh, and by the way. The creator of *Alice in Wonderland*, Lewis Carroll, once said:

'Don't live a life full of regret. You'll never regret taking a chance and betting on yourself.'

Chapter 2
The Camel's Back

B ack in the '70s and '80s I was a prolific 'letter to the editor' person, even though I needed a stamp and an envelope back then—it was before the internet.

> You may or may not remember but former Vice President Al Gore, in 1999, was famously misquoted when he said that he 'took the initiative creating the internet'? Well, just to set that record straight, he really was not trying to say he invented it but he did, in fact, introduce a bill back as early as 1991 that many say helped lead to the internet boom. Also to his credit, in 2012, he was among one of the first inducted into the Internet Hall of Fame for being a Global Connector. Just saying.

I wrote all these letters because I wanted a voice addressing what I thought were limitations or even errors in the way health was being viewed. And it was a way for me to tell if anyone was interested in listening. If it got printed, someone thought it was worth mentioning. It was encouraging because most of what I wrote got "published".

At first, most of my ranting was about the government's dietary recommendations—even before the food guide pyramid and its many iterations. As we now know, the government's recommendations were greatly influenced by the food lobbies and what they wanted Americans to eat **and not what was necessarily best for our health.**

But the one topic I wrote most about was hydrogenated oils, more commonly called trans fats. Back then we were told to eat margarine, cool whip and cheese whiz to save our hearts. Contrary to that, I was telling everyone how much healthier they would be just eating butter, real cream and real cheese. That was the '80s and it took until 2018 for the FDA to ban trans fats completely. They finally had to admit that trans fats were actually creating **more** heart disease, not less. Most shocking to me was that the American Heart Association was also telling everyone to use margarine and nothing I could say to them seemed to make any difference. I mean, I knew margarine was bad, so why did they not know?

Our problem in the US is that too much of the advice coming down from the government is not necessarily in our best interest but instead because of **special interests**. I'm not going to list for you all the potential "bad things" that slide by, and there are many. BTW (by the way) please take the time to search something like 'worst FDA approved foods.' **READ LABELS** and if you can't pronounce it, don't buy it and/or look it up.

Now let's see how the camel can be a powerful metaphor for your health.

Some camels can carry nearly 1,000 pounds, maybe more, but the truth is enough is enough, and eventually there is the proverbial 'straw that breaks the camel's back'. In reality, I think the camel would seriously spit in my face and give me a swift and painful kick way before its back broke.

So what's a camel's back got to do with our health? Well, it means we can eat fast food every now and then and that's just fine. We might be fine with a prescription here and there, but when we start needing prescriptions to try to alleviate the side effects of our prescriptions, it might be time to look at other alternatives. Or we might like a drink of alcohol every now and then and that's fine, but if it's every day and in excess it's taking its toll. I have caffeine and simple sugar in my diet, but I know that in excess they are harmful.

So as we add on more and more of these things that are not really good for us in unreasonable amounts, the problem arises for us just like it could for the camel. Only what it can cause for us can be much more problematic than dropping a load of straw on the ground.

A note about prescription drugs: There is no doubt that prescription drugs have been of great benefit to many. Certainly insulin has made a better quality of life possible for the 12.5 million Americans with type 1 diabetes.

But you know, the strange thing is that the camel, who is supposedly not as smart as we are, wouldn't overload its own back - even if it could - but we do overload ourselves all the time and by choice.

Inherently most of us know what's good for us and much of what's not, so maybe it's just that we're not keeping track—or do we not want to know? I guess it could be that denial thing. We just don't want to admit it. Or could it be that procrastination thing. We're going to get around to doing better—tomorrow. Of course let's not forget rationalization.

As I said previously, denial can be a good thing, such as when we need to temporarily remove ourselves emotionally from a painful or stressful situation. But I think in the case of what we consume, we may have heard that it's not good for us but we don't bother to find out why and, that way, we can use denial to keep it on the menu.

Rationalization, by its nature, is telling yourself a lie, or at least a half truth, so you can do what you want to do. For me, my favorite thing was to rationalize drinking alcohol more often and sometimes in greater quantities than I knew was particularly good for me.

I'd tell myself things like:
- o It's been a tough day and I deserve it.
- o I can't possibly let her/him drink alone.
- o I read somewhere that it's good for me.
- o I'm healthy so it's okay.
- o My favorite - there's hardly anything left in the bottle.
- o I'm on vacation.

So what is the last straw and what causes it?

Honestly, if I knew the definitive, end all answer, I'd be a genius and there could be no sick people. But what I do know for sure is that our bodies are meant to be healthy and that's their default setting. **So when we keep doing things TO our bodies – and not FOR our bodies – then our very intelligent inner self sends us warnings, some subtle and some not.**

Like:
- o Upset stomach
- o Headache
- o Rash
- o Sore throat
- o Back ache
- o Nausea
- o Dizziness
- o Brain fog
- o Memory loss
- o Heart problems
- o Joint pain
- o Shortness of breath

At the rate technology is progressing, before long our cars will be calling us on our phones to tell us they're having a problem, but back in the old days it was different. There were those little lights along the dashboard near the speedometer that came on if we should attend to the oil, temperature or battery. Much like some of the warnings I listed above, those lights only told us there might be a problem but not exactly what it was or the cause. So, when I did speaking engagements back in the '80s and '90s, I liked to use the car and its lights as an example because they helped me to illustrate how silly we could be with our personal health warnings.

I would ask the audience if they would consider it to be a good idea when they saw one of those warning lights come on to just put a piece of tape over it ('I can't see you!') and keep driving as if nothing was wrong. Everyone naturally would say, 'No, that would be stupid!'

I'd say, 'Yea that would be a bit crazy when you knew your car was just trying to tell you that something might be wrong.' I mean, you knew you might be risking something serious, you could mess up your car; it might have to go into the shop or worse—cost you lots of money!

I guess you know where I am going with this. Don't you? If you compare your body to a car, which one is more important? I know that's a tough question for some, but really, which one should we take the best care of? Our body, of course!

So look back at the previous list. They are all warnings but instead of heeding them we tend to 'put tape over them'.

Like:

- o Upset stomach – Nexium®
- o Headache – Aspirin, Tylenol®
- o Rash – Cortisone cream
- o Sore throat – Vick's® Throat Lozenge
- o Back ache – Icy Hot®
- o Nausea – Pepto Bismol®
- o Dizziness – Dramamine

You get the idea, but what do they all have in common?

Is it just because it's what everyone else is doing or is it just easier than having to figure out why we feel this way or that way? Or maybe we don't know we should question why because, again, it's what everyone else is doing.

But in the end, don't we really just want to feel better? Of course, I'm pretty sure I've used many of the above at least once. But that's the whole point—once! Okay maybe a few times, with the exception of aspirin, which I do use to reduce inflammation when working out at the gym. But where the unhealthy things we do to ourselves are concerned, it's a question of **how unhealthy** and/or **how long?** If we do something that's very bad for us, leading to, say, a drug overdose, we can die on the spot. For most, however, it's those subtle things we keep repeating day after day and then year after year until the damage starts to really show up. Things like:

o   Artificial flavors and colors.

o   Chemical detergents.

o   Fluoride in water and other sources, almost all of Europe does not allow it to be added to drinking water. It is a toxic byproduct of industry but then it's added to our water. Definitely check that one out for yourself. BTW, common filters will not remove fluoride from your water. Fluoride, like lead, is what's called a "dissolved solid" and requires reverse osmosis to remove it.

o   Mercury in fish. Shark, swordfish, tilefish, mackerel and tuna have the highest levels. Certified tilapia, salmon, cod and smaller (shorter life) fish in general are the safest.

o   Air pollution.

o   Food preservatives.

o   Some cosmetics.

o   Refined vegetable oils like soybean, corn, cottonseed and canola. Better choices are olive oil, coconut oil and avocado oil.

o   Margarine that is made from one or more of the aforementioned refined oils and can still contain trans fats as long it contains less than 0.5 grams per serving.

o Cooking sprays could be nearly 100% trans fats because they manipulate the serving size. A serving is ⅓ *of a second spray* or 0.3 grams, but can we really spray for only ⅓ of a second? You'd have to be able to push that button 180 times in one minute. Not likely!
o Processed meats. Instead choose meats without additions like nitrites, MSG and large amounts of salt.
o Processed cheese. Instead choose real cheese.
o Any highly processed food.
o Low-fat yogurts when they have taken out the good stuff and added fake stuff. Many don't really having any beneficial probiotics. Try real full fat yogurt and make sure it is certified to contain probiotics.

You get the idea and it's fine to have any of those things sometimes, but they do add up.

*Our bodies are very resilient but, like the water that cuts into a rock as it flows down the stream, **given enough** time the* **affect turns into an effect.** So keep in mind what's going to produce good effects and what's going to produce bad ones.

When loading the camel for a long journey, it's important to balance the load. Like the camel we need to achieve balance in our body. We want to put in more things into our body that 'lightens it up' and less that 'weighs it down'. Load yourself for a long journey, a stable load for a stable body. By reflecting back on this chapter, you should have a great idea of how to load your camel!

No disease that can be treated by diet should be treated any other way

- Maimonide

What to take away:
- o Pay attention to your creative mind games and play to win.
- o Take good care of your "camel".
- o Remember everything you put into, or onto, your body affects it in some way.

Chapter 3
Your Health Status Quo

How do you think you're doing right now in regard to your health? Do you ever ask yourself that question? If you're one of the nearly 90% of Americans who are fortunate enough to have health insurance, more than likely you're covered for an annual physical. For myself, I love having that checkup so I can be told if everything seems to be running okay It's a good thing but this can be where the 'trouble' begins. I'll get to that in a few minutes.

My grandfather was a doctor and served (as a surgeon) in Sebastopol, France in the Johns Hopkins Medical Unit during WWI and was later my doctor as a small child. All my memories of that time are good, especially of the wonderful peppermint candies he kept on his huge desk. He must have passed on his love of medicine to my father who was then my doctor for my teenage years.

I'm not sure whether I was sickly or just wanted to see my father (he didn't live with us), but when I was very young I tried out everything from measles to pneumonia. I fell off a two-story balcony before I could walk and I accidentally nearly cut off my right thumb at the age of six. I remember having the most awful colds and my father had this machine that would flush out my sinuses. It made me feel great right after he used it, but it didn't last long enough to make it really worth the discomfort of the procedure. But that was back in the old days when I still, sort of, did what I was told.

The first of my two biggest takeaways from those days was all the different cold remedy samples he had in his office. It seemed so cool to me that I could get the boxes of pills for free just because the drug reps would drop them off to promote the pharmaceutical company they worked for. I was trained early to use pills as the answer.

The second one was a lesson in how deeply we can take on stuff in our life. When I went to see my father as my doctor, I would often sit in his office and wait for him. Unfortunately, as I realized later, he had all these pictures on the wall of people with terrible skin problems—he probably got them from another drug rep to promote some cream that was going to make everything alright. Later in life, as an adult, I kept having issues with conditions of the skin. I got bites from Black Widow and Brown Recluse spiders plus ticks, which created some kind of rash that came up if I got into cold water. It took me quite a few years to figure that one out and I still think it lingers a bit.

Bottom line – we are the sum total of our beliefs and experiences.

Probably the best way to assess the quality of our health is to honestly ask ourselves how we feel about our self and our life. Do we have plenty of energy to do all the things we want to do in a day? Do we sleep well? Are we ready to get up when it's time? Are we happy with our weight? Are we getting what we feel is a good amount of exercise each week? Do we think our diet is a good one? **How about YOU?** If you're being honest with yourself and can answer with an emphatic yes to all of the above, you're doing great! My guess is if you're reading this book, your answer is not an emphatic yes and maybe not any kind of yes.

I'm grateful every day that I feel fantastic and have excellent health. When I go to the doctor for my annual checkup, I get fantastic test results, but most Americans don't get totally fantastic test results. The bad results are not, in themselves, bad but just those lights coming on. Unfortunately, many doctors are very quick to offer a drug remedy before testing the waters of lifestyle change or maybe they have become frustrated because they realize that most of their patients won't make the necessary changes to turn things around. I wish more health professionals would embrace the idea of food as medicine and that often a simple food addition or subtraction could be all that's needed to get their patient back on the right track.

By definition, medicine is the science or practice of the diagnosis, treatment and prevention of disease.

Sadly, as I have said, the treatment is too often a drug to make the symptoms go away, which is in no way the prevention of disease but a covering up (tape over the warning light) of an underlying cause. Surely, drugs used for temporary measures can be useful, but from the people I've interviewed, it's apparent that it's much easier to get put on a drug than to get taken off one.

And speaking of medicinal drugs, do your homework. Just because your doctor says they're safe does not make it so. I know those people in all the television drug ads look happy and have beautiful smiles, but don't ignore that sweet voice in the background telling you that taking the drug may damage your liver or kidneys and could be fatal. Oh, and the latest warning they have included is, 'Don't take (whatever the drug is called) if you're allergic to it.' Now, how are you supposed to know you're allergic to it until you ARE allergic to it? Isn't it too late? And what if you were? Find out for yourself what the potential side effects are so that awareness is on your radar. This can be a little tricky because, sometimes, knowing about potentials is how we create them so **just know what is possible and choose to keep in your mind the outcome you want.** And another benefit of doing your homework on the side effects is you may be able to supplement in ways that counteract the harm the drug may be causing.

The value of supplementation doesn't just apply to prescription drugs either; for example, stress uses up B vitamins in the body so if you're under lots of stress try taking a B-Complex supplement. Note, take it as a complex of all eight B vitamins and not just individually. And don't overdo it, remember more is not better. Alcohol and sugar are also big depleters—check them out and know the potential side effects. Here also, if you know you are going to partake of an alcoholic drink consider taking some vitamin C beforehand—it can offset the challenges the beverage of your choice gives to your body.

As I mentioned before, it can be a lot harder to get on a drug than to stop using it. My wife is a highly sought-after medical movement therapist and intuitive; just the other day, one of her clients told her that at his last doctor visit his blood pressure (BP) was 102/62. You might think, *Great, he didn't have high blood pressure* and that might be true if he wasn't nearly 90 years old. She questioned him further only to find he was still on BP medication and his doctor had no plans to change them. You see, according to the Harvard School of Medicine and the National Institute of Health, a person over 70, on BP medication, starts to increase their cardiovascular risks when their corrected BP goes below 130 systolic (the top number). So, in this case, leaving this patient on his BP medication may not have been in his best interest. Instead, it seems this person should have been weaned off his blood pressure medicine.

The point is that we start at a young age developing our approach to health and what it means. Early on it is just given to us based on our parents' belief through what the doctor told them was right. Later in life, we start making the choices, but for the most part those choices are to do what the doctor tells us. And we can't forget the commercials on TV, the ads in magazines and, of course, the internet screaming at us. Let's face it; doctors generally know more about health than the rest of us, so they're the best qualified to diagnose our condition at a given point in time. So by all means keep your doctor or nurse practitioner as your first line for diagnosis.

But do your own research and understand the meaning of what might not be just right. And although the internet is a very useful tool it can be a dangerous place if not used carefully. It's mans nature to seek answers that coincide with what we want to believe, but that can leave us open to taking the first bit of information we find. Always be leery of advice attached to an advertisement because, although the statements may be valid, they are, after all, selling something. In other words don't take the first answer you find and look for those answers that are based on valid research and are not just anecdotal. I will share with you some sites whose info is backed by solid evidence-based research. And even if they back it up with research, it can be worthwhile to read the paper attached to the research if you really want to understand. Remember saying something is clinically proven or scientifically proven may not mean anything regarding whether it will work for you. It could mean only tested on animals or simply tested in vitro, Latin for in glass.

And if your health is not what you want then start picturing yourself with the level of health you do want. Don't just accept where you are with your health unless that's where you want to be. Be open to change.

What to take away:

- o Be honest about where you are with your health status and know where you want to be.
- o Don't blindly follow anyone's advice (even mine) and be your own information advocate.
- o Be aware of what you're putting in and on your body.

Chapter 4
How Rich Do You Really Want to Be?

There are certainly more types of diets out there than I have fingers and toes and they all boil down to quite a few good ones and some not so good ones. But the important thing about choosing a particular diet is that it is just that—a diet. Whether it's the DASH, Ornish, Keto, Paleo, South Beach or Atkins, they are all still diets. And many of these diets are functional, meaning they will produce some special response like weight loss, blood sugar regulation or cancer prevention. While these are all good results to achieve, these diets may be promoting only function over all around balance. I will mention the Keto diet, for example, because it is the big fad today and can mean a weight loss bonanza for many but it can be dangerous for others. It's not a diet that should be stayed on long term because without the proper knowledge it will cause future health problems. It's being studied for its potential benefits for seizure disorders and diabetes and therefore it is, as I have said, functional. It's not the diet for life.

So really, we need to just find a healthy way to eat so we can say, 'This is it, **this is how I eat**.' It's not based on just eating one type of food or causing our body to have some special reaction to magically take off unwanted fat. Problem is that once we've tired of the special diet we were on, what are we going back to? What we really want is the diet we are going to live on and does, for us, what we need. It doesn't need to have a name, but it does need to make sense for us if we want to have *Crazy Rich Health!*

My version of Crazy Rich Health is that I'm presently 6'2", around 152 pounds, muscular, about 11% body fat. It took effort to get in shape but now, at age 68, I'm working towards doing the Murph in 44 minutes or less on Memorial Day 2019.

Now, I put in the disclaimer because my wife just saw an article that stated that the Murph was really for the 20 and 30-somethings. It said it might not be safe for people in their forties or older so maybe check in with your doctor to see what he thinks if you plan to try it.

But I do drink alcohol and I eat ice cream, potatoes, pasta, bananas and maybe a steak here and there on special occasions. I love to make key lime pie, chocolate mousse and mango cobblers and serve them up with plenty of whipped cream or, as special treat, ice cream on a warm cobbler. But I'm sure you must know I don't do any of that in excess. Okay, maybe here and there on a special occasion.

Extra: The Murph Challenge was created in 2014 in honor of Navy Lt. Michael Murphy, a SEAL who died in Afghanistan in 2005 in a battle with the Taliban. That battle later became famous in the Mark Wahlberg movie *Lone Survivor.*

Murphy created the workout that the challenge is now known for, and it's definitely intense. Here's the breakdown:

A 1-mile run.

Easy, right?

Then 100 pull-ups.

OK- it suddenly just got MUCH harder.

Then 200 pushups.

Then 300 squats.

And ANOTHER 1-mile run.

Serious CrossFitters might wear a 20 lb. vest as well. You're allowed to break down the workout into 20 rounds of 5, 10, and 15 but still contiguous. It's designed to be done in less than 75 minutes including rest time. I won't be wearing the vest, at least not the first time I try it. Believe it or not, it's been done in less than 25 minutes. Whaaaaat!

Most Americans are on what is referred to as the:

Standard American Diet (SAD)

According to standardprocess.com, SAD comes from the following statistics:

1. **Processed foods make up close to 70% of the U.S. diet.** Frozen fruits and vegetables count as processed, but this is still a sobering statistic.

2. **Americans spend 10% of their disposable income on fast food.** One in four Americans eats fast food every day. *I'm sure I don't even spend 1%.*

3. **The average American consumes 130 pounds of sugar in a year.** That is equivalent to about three pounds every week per person. *My Note: In caloric terms that's 5,325. And if you don't burn it off as you take it in, that 5,325 means adding 1 ½ pounds of fat per week. But look on the bright side, if you cut that same amount out per week (500 per day) you will lose 1 ½ pounds per week and that's 77 pounds per year.*

4. **More than one third of U.S. adults are obese** (not just overweight) with an estimated associated annual medical cost of $147 billion. Of U.S. children ages 2–19, 17% are considered obese, meaning you have a BMI of 30 or higher. You can check out your BMI at: https://bmi-calories.com/calorie-intake-calculator.html

5. **In the early 2000s, 60% of all American middle schools and high schools sold soft drinks in vending machines.** Fortunately, federal guidelines were established in 2014 to phase out the marketing of soda and other sugar-laden drinks and food during the academic school day. An aside: I was able to get soft drink and snack machines out of the schools my children went to in the '90s.

6. So maybe SAD is you or maybe you're better or worse (I hope not). No matter where you are, let's look at how to get Richer!

Richer Health Basics

o Assess where you are with your health right now.
o Definitely buy a body weight scale. $10.00. Weigh every day at the same time. I think first thing in the morning is best.

- o Maybe even a food scale to measure portion size. $11.00.
- o Fitbits are excellent for tracking calories in and calories out and the cost starts at about $120.00.
- o Or you can get a free calorie counting app. Like MyFitnessPal or MyNetDiary.
- o Keep a Food and Exercise Diary of what you eat and how much you move—Be Honest. Again you can download something free or a simple spiral notebook works.
- o Figure your calorie needs or BMR. Again, go to https://bmi-calories.com/calorie-intake-calculator.html
- o Have a vision of the level of health you want and hold it in your mind. Stop looking at what you may not like about your health and **start imagining the life you will have when you have the level of health you want.**
- o Believe you can do it and stay focused on your course.

What to take away:
- o Get some inexpensive tools—especially that scale.
- o Create your diet, one based on what you are learning in this book, one you want to live with. Of course, be open to treating yourself at times. I sure do.
- o Keep records to keep yourself honest.
- o Don't be SAD.

Chapter 5
Get Rich Quick

I guess the first thing I say to anyone who wants to be healthier is:

- o   Cut out the super processed foods.
- o   Cut way down on added sugar, especially corn syrup and soft drinks. Diet drinks are no better if they contain artificial sweeteners. And they really don't help you lose weight in the long run, unless they happen to be water.
- o   Avoid all-you-can-eat buffets.
- o   Eat at home or something from home most of the time.

It's safe to say that the further food gets from its natural state the less good it is for us and the more harm it does. Added sugar is just calories and unless we just need pure energy right away, it's not doing us any favors. Buffets just mean overeating and that's bad in more ways than just too many calories. I used to love them and I really wanted to get my money's worth, so I made sure I ate at least two days' worth of food.

The good comes from the things that nourish our bodies and the harm comes from the things that tax our body's resources.

Nourish: verb – provide with the food or other substances necessary for growth, health, and a good condition.

Harm: noun – physical injury, especially that which is deliberately inflicted.

Sugar is a required nutrient in the body and is generally our main source of energy on a daily basis. But sugar is a complex thing, and I'm not going to go into monosaccharide, disaccharide and polysaccharide or fructose, glucose and lactose, just to mention a few, because it's not necessary to know about them right here for our purposes. There's plenty of information online if you want to sweeten your knowledge of sugar.

At this point you hopefully have calculated your approximate *stay where you are* calorie needs **BMR**. If not you can go here: Try   https:/bmi-calories.com/calorie-intake-calculator.html.   If you're happy with your current weight then you can just skim through this part. For example, if you are age 45, 5"10", 180 pounds and a fairly sedentary male, your daily calorie need, **BMR**, is about 1,780 and if a female about 1,550. For this example and easy math, let's use 2400 calories per day (more like a 270 lb. male). That's 100 calories per hour your body will process for you and use with no net change in weight. So, basically, if you eat more than 100 calories in an hour and you do nothing to increase your base 100 calorie needs, your body will save them for later. And guess how it does that? Our short-term quick energy is stored in our muscles mostly and our liver next, but if they start to get depleted our fat reserves provide the building blocks to restore the muscles and liver so that you can keep going.

But basically, if our muscles are all happy and our liver is all happy and we don't have any immediate energy need, our body stores any extra energy (from food) as fat. Of course, there are all kinds of complex sugar, hormone and enzyme things going on and you are certainly not just feeding your muscles and liver. There are entire books written about sugar and its role in our health, but in this case my point is that sugar is energy, calories. I talk about it more later but the simpler the sugar the more quickly it will get stored if not used.

If you continue throughout the day to eat more than the 100 calories an hour you need in this example, you are going to increase your *bottom line*–plus your hips, stomach and waist *line*.

Of course, it's not quite as cut and dried as that, nor does it mean that if you eat more than 100 calories you will immediately add on fat. But it does mean that, on a daily basis, if you regularly eat more calories than you need you will gain weight by storing fat.

But again, on the bright side, it does work both ways of course. If you eat fewer calories than you need on a regular daily basis you will lose weight by ridding yourself of stored fat.

Note: your body has to run on something so, although there are plenty of people who say you need to do this special diet or that special cardio, the energy you need has to ultimately come from using up fat stores.

Think about this: a 24 oz. soft drink is about 600 calories of sugar and if that is over and above the food calories you need to take in during the day then that alone will cause you to put on over 1 pound in just six days. And that's a scary 61 pounds in a year. Yikes!

But, as before, if you're not gaining weight and you want to lose some, then by the same process you can lose over 1 pound per week by just cutting that out.

One of the most asked questions I get is, 'If sugar is sugar then why does it matter whether I get my sugar from white bread or whole grain bread, cranberries or cranberry sauce?'

What white bread and cranberry sauce have in common is processing, the white bread has been stripped of nutrients and fiber. The cranberries have gone from a 50-calorie super food to a 400-calorie sugar food, which is miles away from the original fruit.

Remember the 100 calories an hour thing? What if I told you that by eating whole grain bread instead of white bread you got to s-t-r-e-t-c-h out the digestion time and reduce the net calories? Well, that is exactly what I'm telling you. The more complex, whole grain bread with its fiber intact not only takes more time to convert to storable sugar but also requires more energy from your body to digest. It's the same for a protein breakfast as opposed to a carbohydrate breakfast. What that means is if you start your day with protein, you'll not be hungry as soon because of the slower digestion time. This slower digestion and longer lasting feeling of satiety (from the Latin satis meaning enough) applies to all complex foods over their processed counterparts. Again, there are many other factors involved in these processes, but we don't need to get caught up in those for this example.

Same with the cranberries, one cup of fresh cranberries has about 4.6 grams of fiber, which is almost 20% of the daily recommended amount. And, of course, cranberries have an incredible amount of antioxidants to fight off all kinds of things like free radicals, which I'll tell you about a bit later.

Of, course cranberry juice cocktail has no fiber, no natural vitamins and more sugar than a can of cola per equal serving.

Those are just a couple of examples, but the point is that you want to add more whole foods to your diet and take away as many stripped down foods as you can.

Whole Foods:
Foods full of nutrients and preferably fresh with nothing added. Like:
- Broccoli
- Spinach
- Peas
- Green Beans
- Lettuce **(not iceberg)**

- Cucumbers
- Potatoes (in moderation)
- Brown Rice
- Barley
- Legumes
- Carrots
- Asparagus
- Kale
- Collards
- Tomatoes
- Avocados
- Apples
- Oranges
- Lima Beans
- Brussels Sprouts
- Beets and Their Greens
- Unprocessed Fish and Meats
- Olive Oil

You get the idea. And just Google 'easy, healthy ways to cook them.' Raw is good, too, for most of them.

Not Whole Foods:

- Stove Top Stuffing
- Sweetened Juices
- Soft Drinks (including diet)
- Store Bought Pies and Cakes
- Frozen Pizza
- Chips
- Bleached White Flour
- Cookies and Crackers
- Processed Cooking Oils (especially corn and soybean)
- Processed Meats, Vienna Sausage, Fish Sticks (or other breaded meats)

o Processed Cheese

For the most part, if we stay away from the inner part of the store and shop the perimeter, we can avoid much of the processed stuff. And I want to say again that having anything from the previous list above is okay now and then. A good rule might be to try to have whole food calories at least 80% of the time with 20% of the time maybe not, to allow for traveling, socializing and eating out.

Oh, and don't forget to drink enough water each day. There are lots of opinions on what is enough, but a good rule of thumb might be half your body weight number in ounces of water. In other words, if you weigh 140 pounds, try to get 70 ounces of pure water or healthy water beverages per day.

What to take away:
> o Whole foods and fiber are your friends and they nourish your body.
> o Processed foods and added sugar are not your friends; they are harmful to your body and lack the nourishment of whole foods.
> o Remember, anything unnatural you take into your body uses up your body's reserves and may just *overload your camel.*
> o If dieting, calculate you calorie needs and eat less each day. Try to vary the difference to keep your body guessing and you'll do better. Remember every 3500 calories cut out means about 1 lb. lost.

Chapter 6
Long-Term Investing

When I was in my 20s, I didn't have a clue about how to eat or even why I should care. I guess I probably first started to care (at least about my weight) when I reached about 225 pounds. Even though that qualified me as obese, I would still joke about it saying I looked like this sort of chubby faced singer (Wayne Newton) but I didn't have his money. I guess I thought that money would make me not care about my weight. BTW, Wayne was a big deal in Las Vegas starting back in the '70s and he's still going today.

Like I said, I got to be 225 pounds and I did it by eating, most evenings, two grape jelly and Jif peanut butter sandwiches on Wonder white bread washed down with Golden Guernsey (extra fat) whole milk (a snack of over 1000 calories). I bet I would just love the taste of that even today; but I know the price now and by that I mean the detriment to my health. Although the "price" today is different it is still questionable. Back then, they used partially hydrogenated oil/trans fats to stabilize the peanut butter so it could last longer and be 'Creamy Jif'. As I mentioned before, that stuff was finally banned (limited) because it did the opposite of what it claimed to help.

But today these types of butters are still not all real and that's because it's still more important to make the product sell well, and most people don't want to have to stir up their peanut butter to keep the oil mixed in. I just keep mine in the refrigerator and that seems to do it. What they and many, many other products now use is something called interesterified oil. (I think it's funny that the word terrified is almost in it.) Already one small study finds that it does, in the body, many of the bad things that the now banned trans fats did and that was to raise LDL (L for lousy), the bad, cholesterol and lower HDL (H for healthy), the good, cholesterol. For me, I believe I'll just avoid anything with that in it until it has been studied a bit more.

In the long run, **to have a full, healthy life**, it's a good idea to take good care of our bodies. Everyone reaches the point in their lives when they stop feeling invincible and start thinking about their health. But as Ben Franklin might have said, it would be better to avoid the 'fire' instead of having to put it out later.

And that 'fire' could be diabetes, heart disease, high blood pressure, high cholesterol, liver disease, kidney disease or cancer to name some of the big ones. Or maybe life just seems harder all of a sudden because you have less energy due to the stress placed on the body.

So let's examine a bit more some of those things that help to make us *Crazy Rich Healthy* and some of those that steal our riches.

The things that nourish!

Our bodies, just like our cars, need certain things to work properly. In the case of your car, it's basically gas, oil, brake fluid, transmission fluid water and anti-freeze. Oh yea, windshield washer fluid because **we want to see clearly where we're going in life.**

Of course, our bodies are, again, certainly more complex than a car but they do need maintenance. We are replacing nearly 300 billion cells per day so it pays to care about the building blocks. For us it comes down to fuel—food, air, sunlight, water and exercise. And if we use quality materials and committed efforts we can expect our bodies to run well and last for a very long time.

What to feed yourself:

Breakfast, at least five days a week, I like to think of it as a really nourishing - easy to make, *be sure I do something good for* *my body* - thing to do. So try having a shake/smoothie with a really good multivitamin. A great shake is Orgain® Organic Protein™ (chocolate or vanilla) 150 calories, 21 g protein, 3 g net carbs and 7 g fiber. Mix it with water or unsweetened almond milk. Also Garden of Life® Raw Organic Protein (vanilla) 110 calories 22 g protein, 2 net carbs, 1 g fiber plus probiotics. Both are tasty, especially with almond milk, and available on Amazon, at Costco and I'm sure many other places. They are both vegetable protein, free of soy and **do not cause the inflammation of animal protein**. I like adding some fruit, part of an avocado and different seeds like chia, sesame and flax (grind the flax to a meal for digestion).

Weekends, breakfast usually consists of eggs on whole grain bread and some kind of uncured meat or a crab cake. But like the weekdays, we are making sure we get protein in the morning. BTW, eggs really are not bad for you and can even increase your good, HDL, cholesterol.

Lunch is the one that gets so many of us in trouble for many reasons. We don't have our refrigerator with us that we **may have** stocked with healthy choices. We often end up eating out and that is dangerous. I like iced tea so I go into McDonald's two or three times per week and get a sweet tea with three pieces of lemon. Of course, I have mostly unsweetened tea with a touch of sweet to take the edge off. BTW, they brew the tea and use cane sugar, not a tea powder, and no corn syrup. But the reason I brought it up is because as I go inside to pick up my order, I get to smell fries, burgers and see those incredible pictures they flash up on the multiple screens. On a regular basis, these days, I'm probably 98 out of 100 resisting any add-ons. I make my order mobile so it's already paid and I don't even need to go to the register to hear, 'Would you like fries with that?'

And speaking of those pictures of the huge, juicy burgers dripping with cheese, I was mean a couple of times way back when I ordered a cheeseburger; I opened it up, took it back to the register and asked if they got my order wrong. The poor employee said, 'No, that's the right thing.'

So I held it up and pointed to the burger and then to the picture that advertised the burger and said, 'Does that look like the same thing to you?'

She replied, 'Well, not exactly.'

Exactly! Maybe if the pictures were true to life it would be a little easier to resist the temptation. Luckily for me, in the 10 years of my life that I was not self-employed I really couldn't afford to eat out all the time so I took my lunch. Generally it was chicken salad or egg salad on whole wheat bread (grains are best organic or at least non GMO). If bread does not work for you, just have salad without the bread. These days there are plenty of non-flour chips that are delicious and loaded with fiber and protein.

A note; don't fall for the idea that gluten-free on its own means healthy because some of the things that processors use to make "gluten free tasty" are pretty bad for you. Read the label. And remember, if you don't have any low blood sugar issues, skipping lunch is okay, too, and a good way to burn fat and do body maintenance because it's a kind of a fast. More on that later.

Dinner is my favorite meal of the day, and it is usually five days a week seafood, one day vegetable protein and one day meat, usually organic chicken. And as I said before, we have an occasional steak. I've been a chef many times in my life and cooking is my way of relaxing. It's easy to bake a piece of fish (use parchment paper in your baking dish for easy cleanup) and cook up a 'mess of greens' or some broccoli. Something green. If you need to lose weight or you don't want to gain, don't overdo the pasta, rice, bread or potatoes; in fact, try leaving the starches out five days a week.

And a note: If you can afford it and have access, I believe there is great value in choosing organic. Look up a list of best choices of where to spend your organic money by searching 'best foods to eat organic' for more details.

Charles Harwood

What to avoid:

As I alluded to earlier, your body has to process or at least **attempt** to process everything you give it. And although most of what I eat is totally good for me and really nourishing, I will eat an Egg McMuffin. The Canadian bacon contains sodium nitrite, something that is in plenty of processed meats because it helps them to retain color and freshness, but in excess it's linked to cancer. So why do I eat it? Well, because it tastes good, I don't do it very often and it's probably the only food that I have that contains nitrites.

But it's that camel again. One of the responses your body has to 'invaders' is the creation of **free radicals**. Free radicals are atoms or molecules that are highly reactive with other cellular structures because they contain unpaired electrons. **Free radicals can cause damage** to parts of healthy cells such as proteins, DNA, and cell membranes by stealing their electrons through a process called oxidation, which effectively leads to the death of that cell.

Antioxidants are molecules that **can** safely interact with **free radicals** and terminate the chain reaction before vital molecules are damaged. Although there are several enzyme systems within the body that disarm **free radicals**, the principal antioxidant nutrients are **vitamin** E, beta-carotene, **vitamin** C, and selenium. Check on food sources and if you don't think you're getting enough then look for a good supplement. Check the resource chapter.

And remember, supplements are just that, they're meant to supplement our diet and not be our diet. And keep in mind, like food, when it comes to supplements **more is not always better.** While on the subject of supplements let me say that there are many opinions about which ones, how much and whether we even need them. Many health professionals will say that if we eat a good diet then we don't need to supplement. In my opinion, that would only be true if:

   o   We had no stress in our life.

o We only ate healthy foods with no additives, no chemical residues and close to all the nutrients they had when they were still living.
o We drank an adequate amount of pure water each day. Avoid added fluoride if possible—again, look it up; fluoride is harmful.
o We got plenty of exercise. More on that later.
o We took no medications.
o We breathed only fresh, clean air.

So raise your hand if you pass on all of the above.

Okay, I only see one hand out of 100, and I believe that's the monk from the Himalayan monastery. Thanks Jungney!

We all know it's pretty hard to be "perfect" every day in the way we nourish our bodies and minds so it's not likely that we'll give ourselves all we need to be the best we can.

I take a natural multivitamin, an immune system supporter (Nutriferon) that promotes the production of Interferon and Ubiquinol (the active form of CoQ10), which promotes energy production, antioxidant support and cardiovascular health. Also I have vitamin C, 1-2000 mg, twice a day.

I add several herbs, seeds, vegetable powders and vitamins to my smoothie on the weekdays like turmeric, beet root, ginkgo biloba, chia seeds, sesame seeds, flax seeds (again meal, not the seeds with flax, because your stomach will not easily break them down). A coffee grinder works great if you want to buy the less expensive seeds rather than flax meal; besides, the seeds keep better than the meal.

Make it a challenge to find what will enhance **your** health and add them to a morning smoothie. Get organic if possible. I love the Nutri Bullet but you can get a digital blender for $9.00 at Walmart.

What to take away:
- Keep in mind the things that are going to nourish your body like organic whole foods.
- Know what the things are that will make your body have to work harder and cause cell damage.
- In the case of our bodies, "hard work" means our body is constantly trying to do repair.
- Remember that no matter how well you eat, it's probably a good idea to add some supplements, at least a food-based natural multi, to your diet. Unless you plan to go live with Jungney.

Chapter 7
Diary of My December 2018 Vacation

At the point of writing this part of the book I'm on vacation in Florida with my wife. We have been here for about 10 days and it is pretty interesting in relation to this book. We are back home in three days on Christmas Day and so I'll check in with my home bathroom scales to see what I've done with my weight. It will be very interesting to see how many pounds I've put on in what will be 13 days. I'm guessing at this point about six pounds. So if we go back to the example I gave you earlier, I needed to take in 21,000 extra calories. In order to achieve that I ate too much and I consumed too much alcohol.

* * *

It's Christmas Eve now and we head back home tomorrow, compared to my normal self I don't feel all that great. Great is relative, of course, as I know from past experiences that my "not all that great" is someone else's feeling good. The extra weight in my case is obvious because at 11% body fat, six pounds is hard to hide from myself. But that brings up the point that if someone is already overweight it can be hard to notice putting on a pound here and a pound there and I guess that's one way we just keep adding on the weight. And that's why **having a weight scale is so valuable when trying to stay at a weight or lose weight or even gain weight.** Of course, because we flew it was not really convenient to take our scales. I know the first thing I'll do the morning after I return will be to weigh myself to see what the "damage" is. I'll know what I gained and I'll cut back so I get back to the weight and good feeling I had when I left for vacation.

But right now I can feel how my stomach has stretched to accommodate the "feast", a clever design by the creator or evolution, whichever you believe. Our stomach was made to accommodate large amounts of food during times of plenty that we can store as fat. And that surplus fat also signals our body to slow down the metabolism to save our new stores. It's another of the two-edged swords of weight control. I think at first our body thinks that if we are putting on weight all of a sudden we must be heading into some tuff times and there may not be much food so it's slows down the metabolism. On the other hand, if we start to lose weight then at some point our body becomes a little more comfortable with what's ahead and our metabolism starts to speed up. I believe that the metabolism rate sort of levels out around 22-24% body fat for a woman and around 15-17% for a man. Once our body fat level gets much lower I believe our body starts slowing down the metabolism again just in case we are heading for famine.

That slowing down is one of the reasons you just don't see too many people with six-pack abs. You see, we can do all the sit-ups and crunches we want and it will help to give us bigger, stronger muscles, but we'll never have a visible six pack if we have too much fat in the way. So most of our movie heroes have to really work to look like that and, trust me, they don't look like that all the time. Body builders might get their fat level down as low as 3-6% for a competition but they know it's not healthy to stay there long. I won't go into the effects of age, body types and location of fat stores but they do have an effect as well. As they say, "six-pack abs are built in the kitchen." You can check out some pictures at:

https://www.builtlean.com/2012/09/24/body-fat-percentage-men-women/

Keep in mind that most of the people in the photos are 25–30 years old.

* * *

Today is Boxing Day, the day after Christmas. We're home and I weighed in at 159.8 so that's almost 8 pounds. I panicked a bit when the digital readout blipped on 160 as that was a number I'd not seen since probably 2013. Of course I know that a couple of pounds will go away the next day just because my digestive system is just fuller than usual. But how about that warm brownie and vanilla ice cream I had in the Atlanta airport on the way home?

I know I'm full because, last night, once I was in bed, my stomach was talking to me saying, "Are you done yet? Do you really want to stretch me more?" All I know is I was pretty uncomfortable.

* * *

The next morning, my weight went down to 155.4 mainly because I ate my normal diet, which is a lot less bulk and sugar. I probably won't do much more than that until January 2nd when I have no excuses for anything but getting back to normal. Within two or three weeks I plan to be back to the weight I was when I left for vacation.

* * *

So what I took away was that I was still very good at rationalization but there was no denying that I felt less and less my normal energetic self as each day went by and that was just two weeks. The strangest thing I got to thinking was how I was really looking forward to getting back to my normal routine so I could get back to feeling better, but at the same time I continued right on through New Year's Day to do too much of those things that were not going to let me feel normal self. I mean, I could have just stopped the abuse.

Ultimately, it took me until January 7th to really get back on track. I still had the excuse the week before that it was still New Year's week. Really? I'm on it now!

Beginning on the 7th I got myself back into my normal routine of a smoothie on weekday mornings, a very light lunch, if any, and then an early evening fish, vegetable and no starch dinner. It was pretty awesome how the light feeling started to come back and the energy level just shot up. Of course, not having an alcoholic drink every night sure made a big difference in not only taking off the excess weight but also in how good I felt.

The important thing is that I worked hard to get back to the healthy guy I was before I went on vacation. It was not always easy and I sure thought up plenty of excuses to not 'do the right thing'.

In the end, I did it. Yeah me!

Chapter 8
Walking or Weights?

I am forever talking to people at the gym about the value of resistance training. Because I'm very lean I'm always asked, 'Are you a runner?' or, because my shoulders are broad, 'Are you a swimmer?' Truth is I am neither, although I do think that someday I will develop gills or some other way to breathe under water because I do love being in water.

While simply walking daily is probably one of the best things one can do for so many reasons, let's look at some facts. For most people, a cardio session will probably burn more calories than a weight/resistance training session and that is mainly because most people will spend more time in cardio than they do with weight training. They don't tend to push themselves in the weight training. For example, what I see most people (the ones I imagine were in a study I read) do is treat weights like cardio. In other words, they pick up a five-pound weight and do 50 repetitions, which they break up into five sets of 10. And don't get me wrong, that does have benefit but hardly enough to change their muscle composition. You don't want to hurt yourself but find a weight you can only push/move 10 times and do three sets with that. Now you're building muscle. Always warm up with a lighter weight.

And why do you want to build muscle? Glad you asked!
- o If you're trying to lose weight you might burn more calories in the cardio session (see above) but from the muscle-building session your metabolism will be increased for hours afterward and even into the next day. Additionally, the more you increase the amount

of developed muscle in your body the more you raise your resting metabolic rate. Now you can burn more calories while you sleep. I love effortless healthy weight loss.

o Certainly most of us have heard that as we age our bone becomes less dense. This is mainly due to poor diet and inactivity. Weight training puts stress (good stress) on our bones and makes them stronger and denser.

o As you push the weights repeatedly your heart gets better at transporting oxygen, making it stronger.

o You will sleep better because the need for muscle repair causes our body to want to sleep.

o Better brain function is another benefit of weight training. Research has shown that hitting the weights improves cognitive function, especially in older adults.

o Weight training also causes our body to produce those feel good endorphins. We should never underestimate the benefits of looking and feeling great, and seeing those 'mirror muscles' is a big boost to how we feel.

Streamline your cardio by trying HIIT training. HIIT stands for High Intensity Interval Training and it can give you the same or better results as cardio in half the time. A HIIT routine can be done in so many ways and usually includes a combination of resistance and cardio. But when it comes to streamlining cardio and taking less time you can simply increase the intensity/speed of your cardio, but do it for only one minute that way and then revert back to a slower pace, a pace that allows you to easily carry on a conversation. **Of course, I should repeat the disclaimer that you might need to check with you doctor if you are not sure you can push yourself harder.** But if you can do it and you are used to doing 30 to 60 minutes of standard cardio, you can cut that back to 15-30 minutes with the same and even more benefit.

The main thing is to keep moving. We certainly don't need to do hours of cardio every day, just avoid sitting all day. In fact, recent studies have found that those who performed one to two and a half hours of moderate cardio, like a brisk walk, per week scored better on some heart health tests than those doing a greater number of hours. They found that excessive cardio can actually be detrimental, so if you just like spending lots of time at the gym **try cutting back a bit on cardio time and increase your resistance training time.**

I can't talk about weight training and not mention the importance of protein for recovery. You see, if you do push yourself a bit your body needs protein to help your muscles to recover. So, as soon as you can, after a strength workout be sure to take in some lean protein or a protein supplement like the ones I mentioned before. The American College of Sports Medicine recommends between .5 and .8 grams of protein per pound of body weight each day. In other words, if you weigh 130 lbs. you need 65-104 grams of protein per day. And if you are working out strenuously then lean more towards the .8 or more. And another point about protein is that first thing in the morning is a great time to have it because it will keep you satisfied much longer than a simple carbohydrate breakfast.

What to take away:
- o While a daily walk is a really good thing to do, don't forget your muscles.
- o Don't spend hours a day only doing cardio.
- o Building muscle has benefits beyond the workout. It raises your metabolism and strengthens your bones.
- o Protein is essential in building muscle.

Chapter 9
Stretching to the Sun

If you're really going to have a healthy and fit body you need to stretch and 'see the light'.

It's important to not only focus on building muscle and achieving aerobic fitness but also to maintain flexibility.

You may think of stretching as something performed only by runners or gymnasts, but we all need to stretch in order to protect our mobility and independence. A lot of people don't understand that stretching has to happen on a regular basis. It should be done daily.

Why is it important?

Stretching keeps the muscles flexible, strong, and healthy, and we need that flexibility to maintain a range of motion in the joints. Without it, the muscles shorten and become tight. Then, when you call on the muscles for activity, they are weak and unable to extend all the way. That puts you at risk for joint pain, strains, and muscle damage.

For example, sitting in a chair all day results in tight hamstrings in the back of the thigh; that can make it harder to straighten your leg or extend your knee all the way, which can cause pain when walking. Likewise, when tight muscles are suddenly called on for a strenuous activity that extends them, such as playing tennis, they may become damaged from suddenly being stretched. Injured muscles may not be strong enough to support the joints, which can lead to joint injury.

Regular stretching keeps muscles long, lean, and flexible, and this means that exertion won't put too much force on the joints themselves because healthy muscles support a balanced skeleton. The areas critical for mobility are in your lower extremities; your calves, your hamstrings, your hip flexors in the pelvis and quadriceps in the front of the thigh.

While females tend to have tighter quads, males are more prone to tight hamstrings. As a general rule, this is simply due to the difference in pelvic structure and not always the case. Stretching your shoulders, neck, and lower back is also very beneficial. Aim for a program of daily stretches or at least three or four times per week. I do it at least once a day and mostly twice.

If you need help getting started you could look for someone to assess you and tailor a stretching program to fit your needs. If you have chronic conditions such as Parkinson's disease, arthritis, or inflammation, you may want to clear a new stretching regimen with your doctor before you start.

A hamstring stretch will keep the muscles in the back of your thigh flexible.

Try sitting on the floor with your legs in front of you. Gently slide your hands down your legs until you feel a mild to moderate tension in your hamstring. Hold for 30 seconds then assist your lower back by pushing up slowly to return to a seated position.

If getting up from the floor is difficult for you, try this one. Sit slightly forward on a sturdy chair. Put one leg out straight with your heel on the floor. Keep the other leg bent and your foot flat. Lean forward, first supporting yourself on the bent knee then working toward both arms hanging toward the floor. Then repeat on the other leg. This is such an easy one to build into your day anytime you are sitting for a while.

A quadriceps stretch will keep the muscles in the front of your thigh more flexible and less likely to pull on your knee joint causing pain.

Stand with a stable high surface behind you and hold on to something in front. While leaning forward and putting one foot behind you on top of a bar stool or any other prop, slowly bring your torso up to vertical until you feel tension at the front of your thigh in your quadriceps. If you feel a pull in your knee joint, find a lower surface on which to put your foot. If you come up to vertical and do not feel the stretch, either raise the surface behind or tighten your butt muscles to stretch the quad a little more.

You'll find that you'll get an easier stretch each time.

Stretching once a day won't magically give you perfect flexibility. You'll need to do it over time and remain committed to the process. It may have taken you many months, even years, to get tight muscles, so you're not going to be perfectly flexible after one or two sessions. Be patient, it may take weeks to months to get flexible, and you'll have to continue working on it to maintain it.

Stretching tips:

It was once believed that stretching was necessary to warm up the muscles and prepare them for activity. However, mounting research has shown that stretching the muscles before they're warmed up can actually hurt them. When everything is cold, the fibers aren't prepared and may be damaged. If you exercise a little first, you'll get blood flow to the area, and that makes the tissue more pliable and amenable to change. All it takes to warm up the muscles before stretching is five minutes of light activity, such as a walk. You can also stretch after an aerobic or weight-training workout to ease the recovery of the muscles.

Hold stretches for 20–30 seconds. Don't bounce; that can cause injury. You'll feel tension during a stretch, but you should not feel pain. If you do, there may be injury or damage in the tissue. Stop stretching that muscle, and talk to your doctor if you're concerned.

Stretching is so valuable because we just get stuck in repeated positions that we hold over and over. Our bodies end up more and more imprisoned by our tight muscles. Don't you want to be free? Be patient; do it right and you'll get results. Strive to progress, not to be perfect!

For illustrations and videos, the internet abounds with examples. Just search for stretches applicable to your present physical condition and abilities.

Lighten up and get happy!

This is a topic on which I have very definite personal opinions. It appears to me that so many people have become afraid of the sun. To me it's the source of life, but it needs to be respected. Vitamin D is such an important nutrient for our bodies and sunlight on our skin is the best source. Vitamin D is instrumental in the treatment or prevention of so many diseases like:

- o Heart Diseases
- o High Blood Pressure
- o Types I & II Diabetes
- o Bone Health
- o MS
- o Macular Degeneration
- o Arthritis
- o Depression
- o Cancer
- o Alzheimer's

Other benefits include better sleep quality and help with weight loss.

Point is, don't hide from the sun completely **but do avoid being burned.** It only takes a few minutes a day of direct contact with sunlight to boost your vitamin D levels. Also, unlike vitamin D supplements that can be overused, your body won't make more than you need. If you need to take a supplement then it seems that natural vitamin D3 is the best. And when you do need a sunscreen for longer daytime exposure, do your homework because many sunscreens are unsafe.

You see, it's the camel again. If you use sunscreens that have potentially harmful ingredients that may be fine if those are the only harmful ingredients that make it to your body. So when the government sets a GRAS (Generally Recognized as Safe) level for a particular ingredient in a product, like sunscreen, it's for that substance and not for that plus all the others that may already be in or on the body. Together they add up to not be GRAS at all. So use one of the natural zinc-based sunscreens that work just as well or better than ones that will unbalance your camel's load.

If skin cancer is a concern, keep in mind that it's those free radicals again. Oxidative damage from the sun, like from anything else, happens when the free radicals outweigh the antioxidants. If you are going for a day in the sun, taking some antioxidants (vitamins C and E) could be another way to protect your skin from damage.

What to take away:
- o Maintaining flexibility is not only doable but also essential for a long, active life. Even if you've lost flexibility it's not too late to make improvements. Take it slow and be patient.
- o Getting into the sun is so beneficial in so many ways. Be smart about it, but don't forget about it.

Chapter 10
Meet Nocebo and Placebo

Most of us have heard of the placebo effect as it relates to someone getting well because they thought they were taking a medicine when, in fact, it was only a sugar pill. In other words, it shows the value of positive expectation and that's a good thing because we rarely hear of anyone being hurt by positive expectation. I learned about this as a child because my father, as I mentioned, was a doctor starting back in the days when doctors still made house calls. I remember him telling me that so many of his patients did not feel they could get well unless they took a pill, so once he determined nothing serious was afoot, he would give them sugar pills and tell them when to expect to be better. They pretty much always got better, but they still would often say they thought they might need some more pills. Great that they could get "well" without taking some drug with its potential side effects. At his retirement party, I found that some people must have caught on to it and he was affectionately called the Sugar Pill Doctor. I guess since they figured out he was using sugar pills they must have worked out they didn't really need them.

But what is the nocebo effect?

A detrimental effect on health produced by psychological or psychosomatic factors such as negative expectations of treatment or prognosis.

To me the power of the mind and its beliefs is major when it comes to our health, our happiness and our life in general. So often I hear someone making a list of reasons why they can't do something, and for each one I help them release, they come up with another. In other words they **"argue for their limitations"**, like 'I'm too old,' 'I don't have time,' 'I've tried everything and nothing works.' I say if we are going argue to for anything, let's argue for our possibilities.

> *'Whether you think you can or you think you can't – you're right.'*
>
> **- Henry Ford**

Don't argue for your limitations! For me, I'm definitely a 'think I can' kind of guy and I do things all the time that many people would not consider trying and certainly not at my age. My feeling is that the more I ask of myself the more my body provides and because I ask for the limits of a 30-year-old, my body does what it can to meet those demands so I have a better chance of doing what I think I can.

So much has been written about the proven power of positive thinking and expectation, but please, please remember that the power of negative thinking can be just as powerful. Many people have affirmation boards where they post pictures and ideas that they want to become reality in their lives. Looking at them can evoke good feelings, positive emotions and powerful visualizations, which are strong tools for having a healthy and happy life. And we all really know that being positive feels better than being negative, so why do we allow ourselves to be negative? Well, this is where your good friend **FOCUS** can play a big part.

Crazy Rich Health

*The successful warrior is the average man
with laser like focus.*

- Bruce Lee

Ever since an encounter with spontaneously feeling sad back
in the '70s I've been aware of the potential of focus. I'd just come
home from having a fantastic lunch with a good friend at an
eclectic café, it was beautiful day and life was good. But as I sat
down on my front porch to watch the world go by for a few
minutes, I realized I was sad verging on depressed. Those were
not the kinds of feelings that were normally a part of my life and if
they had been, I usually knew why.

Fortunately, I had recently been practicing playing back my
thoughts so I decided to see if I could play back the day with as
much detail as possible. I decided I'd start with arriving at lunch
and go from there.

It was somewhat hot that day (I love hot days) and we sat
outside to enjoy watching those who were passing by. I just love
people and, although I know I can't really peer into their thoughts,
I love imagining what each person might be thinking. I won't go
into the details of lunch but it was great. My friend had an
appointment so we finished lunch and departed separately after a
warm hug goodbye. I, too, had a few stops before heading for
home and one of them was in downtown Richmond, Virginia. I
took the interstate and as I started noticing the string of billboards
visible along the side of the road it made me think of Lady Bird
Johnson (wife of our 36th president, Lyndon Johnson). She had a
pet project that resulted in the Highway Beautification Act of
1965, which, among other things, tried to eliminate the clutter of
billboards.

And then BAM, billboard. I figured out it was a billboard
that had changed my mood. I then remembered I'd seen a
billboard for a charity, *Save the Children*, and on it were these

little children in Africa who were so emaciated that almost every bone in their tiny bodies showed. I didn't think at the time that I had taken on any emotion, but I had tucked it away in my subconscious.

My point is that if we can stay focused in the present moment and pay attention to our thoughts then we stand a chance of not having some random sound, sight or smell stir up something that makes us feel bad then or even days later.

Now, more specifically, in regard to having *Crazy Rich Health*, remember to first do your homework and make good food and exercise choices, choices that **work for you** and not necessarily someone else. Next, have very positive expectations for the results you want from your efforts. Have a clear picture that you hold in your mind of what you and your life will be like when you have achieved your goals. **Don't keep checking in to look at what you may not want. Stay focused on what you do want without condemning what you have now.**

Your life is controlled by what you focus on!

- Tony Robbins

What to take away:
  o Your mind, your thoughts are the real rulers of your life. But **they are** yours so make sure you are a great ruler and only do what's good for the kingdom that is you.
  o Our body is given direction by our beliefs. If we keep telling or reminding our body that it is sick how can we expect to be well?
  o If it is our expectation and focus that all is well and everything we ever wanted is waiting for us it's going to be a great ride whether we reach that specific

destination or not. Life is not about reaching the end, it's about enjoying the trip along the way.

Chapter 11
Review of Key Points

The Mind:

I've always thought that the best way to help those close to me in regard to health is to be a good example. My family and friends know that I'm not a health fanatic, they also know I'm very fit and healthy (although my family jokes that they have mixed opinions about my mental health). And if you're one who wants to be there for others, again, what better way than to be your best?

In this book I've referred to those foods that are good for you and many which are unhealthy, but I believe that the biggest and absolutely most important aspect of *Crazy Rich Health* is what we put in our heads. I know so many people who have all the money anyone could want, every device purported to improve their health, they don't eat anything 'unhealthy' and they have the 'perfect' diet. But they are still sick and they can't seem to get themselves just right. I believe their main "disease" may really exist in their minds and emotions.

I would love you to take away from this book the value of getting control of your thoughts and emotions because, like the previous example, if you don't expect great health it will be hard to have it no matter what you do. Remove fear from your mind about getting this disease or that injury. Remember, don't keep saying, 'I won't get this disease,' or 'I won't have that injury.' Instead have a clear picture in your mind of the health and the life you do want to have and hold **those** thoughts. If you already have a health challenge, still focus on being totally healthy, not being relieved of whatever the challenge may be. Never give something you don't want any attention because **if we want to remove something from our lives it's very hard to do so if we keep thinking about it.**

You don't get rid of a dark room by removing the darkness, you do it by adding the light.

- Charles Harwood

The Food:

Our bodies have evolved over the centuries so that all people don't necessarily thrive on the same diet. However, I don't know of any genetic change that has made us thrive on unnatural foods. We have a relationship with nature and especially that of our indigenous environment. The further we get away from eating natural foods the unhealthier we'll become. It's encoded in our body to recognize unnatural substances and to therefore try to rid itself of them. And while our body is very good, in the short run, at defending us from invaders, that defense still uses up our body's reserves and damages our cells.

Certainly, genetics plays a part in how easy or how difficult it might be for us to keep our weight in a healthy range. That being said, a very small percentage of the population has that kind of challenge when it comes to losing weight. If that's truly their desire and they keep focused on the task, they, too, will lose weight because, as I've said, **it's physically impossible not to lose weight if you burn more calories than you take in.** When someone says, 'I can't lose weight, I've tried everything and nothing works,' then I say, 'Be honest, keep a food and calorie diary and get some exercise.' I also hear, 'I hardly eat anything but I still can't lose weight.'

Let me give you this analogy, which comes from the opposite side of weight balance but, as I've said, it works both ways. Still, I think you'll get my point. Let's say you want to drive 100 miles in your car that gets 25 miles to the gallon; how far do you think you will get if you only have one gallon of gas? You do the math!

Point is, if you've (hopefully at this juncture) figured your BMR and its 2,000 and if you only put in 1,500 calories' worth of fuel for the day, you'll eventually be unable to keep going—unless you have some extra fuel somewhere! Of course, if you're overweight you know where you're keeping that extra fuel. I'm not going into the details of where the energy comes from if you're underweight and have zero body fat because that's more than you need to know right here.

Let's go back to the car again for another analogy. When we're pumping in the gasoline, there's that neat little coil of wire near the end of the gas nozzle that tells the gas pump to cut off because it's sensed the tank is full. Of course, we wouldn't try to force in more fuel than our car needs at the time and just let it spill all over the ground would we, especially if we're smoking? Besides, we'd be throwing away money.

More than likely, if we're fairly overweight, we probably broke our "spring" or we're just ignoring it, but I've told you how to get a rough idea of how much fuel you need—so stop overfilling your tank, *especially if you're smoking.* Besides, you'd be throwing away money and if you keep it up *(especially the smoking),* there's a statistically very good chance it will cost you even more later on. I think you know what I mean.

> *"Eating unhealthy food may seem a reward to the mouth, but it's definitely punishment to the body"*
>
> **- Charles Harwood**

Back in the 1990s most grocery stores carried about 7,000 different items and even that seemed a lot of variety. Today, the average grocery carries 40-50,000 different food items.

Unfortunately, in a study that ran from 2000 to 2013 it was found that Americans spend more than 60% of their food dollar on highly processed foods. That's understandable since probably 95% of that difference between the 7,000 in the '90s and the 50,000 of today would have to be processed foods. Let's face it; there were not too many new vegetables, meats, fish or poultry created in that time. Not surprisingly, incidences of obesity, diabetes, and many cancers have also increased over that same period. Obesity alone has increased 60% and I am quite sure the increased use of highly processed foods is responsible for most of those increases and so many more.

The Exercise:

Just as we need fuel to operate our bodies, we must also have an **equal amount** of demand for the fuel. I've given you the tools to know how much fuel you need so let's look again at the best ways to use it.

When you calculated (I just know you have now) your BMI, you found out the amount of food you needed for your normal day. But unless you're a construction worker or a UPS™ driver you'll probably need to find a way to do something that pushes you some, builds, or at least maintains, your muscle and something that elevates your heart rate to keep that muscle strong as well.

As I have said, I am a huge fan of resistance training. It can be done using machines or, if you're comfortable, free weights are even better. The reason I make sure part of my exercise is resistance training and not just cardio is because the benefit of a muscle building session can last for more than a day by keeping our metabolism up. Cardio, of course, does raise our metabolism, but that benefit pretty much ends as soon as we stop running or step off the elliptical, bike or treadmill. Two to two and a half hours per week is adequate so think heart health not calorie burn. Thirty minutes to two hours of resistance training twice a week can do it for you as well. Give yourself at least 48 hours of recovery time for your muscles to repair and grow.

Chapter 12
Closing Thoughts

Intermittent Fasting:

Intermittent fasting is an umbrella term for various eating protocols that cycle between a period of fasting and non-fasting over a defined period. It is an alternative to long-term calorie restriction and it can produce weight loss as well.

One example would be to eat not more than 500 calories for a woman and 600 calories for a man two days per week. You would eat normally the other five days.

Another example might be what's called a 24-hour fast and you might do it once or twice per week. So you basically might finish your dinner and then not eat again (no calories) until dinner the next day.

Additionally, don't be afraid to just skip a meal whenever you feel like it. Of course, if you have blood sugar related issues ease into it or check with your health professional if you need to.

Of course, an obvious bonus is that if you do the 24-hour fast, for example, and you normally consume 500 calories between dinner and dinner the next day, you will lose one pound every seven times you do the fast. In other words, if you have stabilized your weight so that you are neither gaining nor losing weight but you are still carrying more than you would like, it's a simple way to take it off.

What are the potential benefits of fasting?

1. Promotes Blood Sugar Control by Reducing Insulin Resistance
2. Promotes Better Health by Fighting Inflammation

3. May Enhance Heart Health by Improving Blood Pressure, Triglycerides and Cholesterol Levels
4. May Boost Brain Function and Prevent Neurodegenerative Disorders
5. Aids Weight Loss by Limiting Calorie Intake and Boosting Metabolism
6. Increases Growth Hormone Secretion, Which Is Vital for Growth, Metabolism, Weight Loss and Muscle Strength
7. Could Delay Aging and Extend Longevity
8. May Aid in Cancer Prevention and Increase the Effectiveness of Chemotherapy

And on top of all of that, you give your digestive system a rest, which it really appreciates. Your body can use upward of 30% of its energy reserves to carry out digestion and absorption. Move some of that energy to body repair instead of digestion.

You can get more info on this at:
https://www.healthline.com/nutrition/fasting-benefits.

How about Meditation?

Even though I meditate regularly I still get the same picture in my mind of a serene person in Lotus Position whenever I hear someone say the word meditation. Or I might even picture some mysterious monk in a cave in deep contemplation. Not sure where I got that one.

So what are the benefits of meditation? The main benefit, which then leads to so much more, is just to learn to relax. That relaxing, that calming of the body and mind can:

o Lower blood pressure
o Improve blood circulation
o Lower heart rate
o Decrease perspiration
o Slow the respiratory rate
o Decrease anxiety

- o Lower blood cortisol levels
- o Increase feelings of well-being
- o Decrease stress
- o Deepen relaxation

So how do you do it? Well, you don't have to have the cool looking very comfortable clothes that spring up in my mind and definitely no cave.

Start by sitting or lying comfortably on the floor or on a mat *but definitely not on your cat.* Sorry, couldn't resist Dr. Seuss. You can even lie on your bed, although you may just fall asleep, which is not really a bad thing if you have the time.

Close your eyes and if you are lying down you could even put some very comfortable material over your eyes.

Don't try to control your breath; simply breathe naturally.

Pay attention to your breath and how the body moves with each inhalation and exhalation. Notice the movement of your entire body as you breathe. Observe your chest, shoulders, rib cage, and belly. Simply focus your attention on your breath without controlling its pace or intensity. If your mind wanders, return your focus back to your breath. Maintain this meditation practice for two to three minutes to start, and then try it for longer as it gets easier. You will find after some time you will definitely look forward to it.

There are so many types and styles of meditation but I'll tell you about two that are simple.

The first is Concentration or Focus Meditation, which involves focusing on a single point. This could entail following the breath, as in the example above, repeating a single word or mantra, staring at a candle flame or listening to a repetitive sound. Since focusing the mind is challenging, if you are a beginner you might meditate for only a few minutes and then work up to longer durations. In this form of meditation, you simply refocus your awareness on the chosen object of attention each time you notice your mind wandering. Rather than pursuing random thoughts, you simply let them go. Through this process, your ability to concentrate improves.

The second is a Mindfulness Meditation where you are encouraged to observe wandering thoughts as they drift through the mind. The point is not to get involved with the thoughts or to judge them but simply to be aware of each mental note as it arises.

Through mindfulness meditation, you can see how your thoughts and feelings tend to move in particular patterns.

Once I got good at this one while being still, I thought I would see how it went while going through my day. I still have to make a choice to be that way in my mind, but all I really have to do now is slow down, breathe, and focus anytime during my day, of course not while driving or operating dangerous equipment. I love following where my mind goes and noticing how it got there.

The value of meditation, learning to relax and be in the moment, if only for a few minutes a day, is huge. It can really help you to get in touch with yourself and your life. And the better your relationship with yourself, without the shouting going on in your head, the better your health, your happiness and your life in general will be.

These statements have not been evaluated by the Food and Drug Administration. This information is not intended to diagnose, treat, cure or prevent any disease.

Appendix

The four following excerpts are from the teachings of Christian, the main character in my novel *Earthmaster - First Sight*. Besides being a super human, he's a teacher. He teaches his students lessons called The Postures and there are nine of them. Although the name sounds like he's teaching how to stand up straight, in this case it's the other definition of posture: *a particular way of dealing with or considering something; an approach or attitude.* It's the way he's learned to approach life. BTW, they are the way I approach life myself and it's working very well for me.

I've only included the first four Postures because Christian has yet to speak of the other five. They will be revealed in books two and three of my Earthmaster Trilogy.

Posture #1 - Desire: It's the fuel of life!

There are two very important things to keep in mind. First, make sure your desire is for something new to come into your life and NOT to change something that is already there. It's possible to be satisfied with where you are and still move toward to something different. For example, if you're sick, don't desire getting rid of the ailment but instead see your future life with a totally healthy body. Trust me on that, it will be clearer as you move through the Postures. Second, you should decide with your brain what you want but then *let the desire come from your heart!* How you feel about what you want, your emotions, is so much more important than what you think. Besides, the heart, unlike the mind, is not subjective so the heart is more likely to lead you down a path of success.

One more note, which will ultimately apply to all of the Postures. Thoughts really are things! Science is a little behind on wanting to come right out and say it, but Nobel Prize winning physicists Albert Einstein and Max Planck both seemed to believe so and you would be wise to do the same.

You would be wise to know what you want in life and definitely know why. There's no right or wrong thing to want and most people just follow along with the pack and, for the most part, want what their parents, friends or peers want or wanted, and that's okay. But that kind of desire is usually not even conscious, meaning you just go through the motions of being the same as everyone else. That sameness does not generate the extra energy needed to go from mundane to extraordinary.

In order to break out of the pack, it takes a strong desire to be something or someone different. All the great people of history had to want more, to be more and make a difference. And I don't mean necessarily more money or more things. I mean, they knew they didn't want to go through life with a "business as usual" scenario. The status quo is really pretty boring but it can be easy, so that it is the route most taken. To progress through the Postures it is important to desire more than your neighbor. Again, not to be richer or better than your neighbor but to stretch yourself and see what your limits are. Don't be afraid to have big desires either, use your imagination and go for something great. You may have to start with the proverbial "baby steps", but as you start having successes, you will have the confidence to desire bigger and bolder things in your life. The further you reach the more the Universe will send the inspiration and energy to make your desires a reality.

And write down what you desire with as much detail as you can so that it's easy to see in your mind's eye. Imagine what your life would look like if those desires were realized. Keep modifying your list, fine-tuning it, painting a clearer, more vivid picture of your desire. It's important to know why you want something in your life and for most people it's because they think it will make them happier. I love this quote and what it says in this regard.

"The reason you want every single thing that you want is because you think you'll feel really good when you get there. But, if you don't feel really good on your way to there, you can't get there. You have to be satisfied with what is while you're reaching for more."

- Abraham

Posture #2 - Belief:

Remember! If you want to achieve something beyond the "norm" then what is possible in your life has to come from what you believe is possible. It's not likely that you're going to hope for something that you don't think can be. This means you will need to give up some of the things you presently believe are true if they conflict with what you now want to believe. I call that **suspension of belief.** This does not mean you decide to believe you can fly and so you unbelieve that you can't, thereby jumping off a building. Start with flying up first!

But like your desires, your beliefs should stretch you and the more you stretch the more you can create. You might decide to believe that you can have a radically better body and great health and one day you realize that you do. That belief worked in a couple of ways. First, you programed yourself through your thoughts to make choices that supported your belief. And second, those projections of your mind and heart really are things. Consciousness is the building block of the Universe that connects us all, constantly creating our world and adding to the world around us so if we keep thinking the same thoughts it becomes more possible for those things to be in our life.

But please remember, your beliefs can help you or hurt you, it's your choice and you make that choice by the predominant thoughts on your mind and the feelings in your heart. Like desire, your beliefs should be fashioned in ways that support what you want and **NOT what you don't want.** Imagine a future where what you want to believe already exists.

And a very important note about your desires and beliefs coming to fruition: Don't keep checking in to see if you're there yet, just give it time. You see, because everything is really just energy, you may have already done all you need to do to bring it to fruition; in fact, others may even see it before you do. More about that later...

And speaking of others, what you choose to believe may be in conflict with what others believe so I would advise that you don't always share. You will ultimately share with others by your result. Mass consciousness is a strong force by its number but it's weak in its focus and resolve. You see, unwavering focused belief is at least 10 times stronger than belief that just rose out of following the pack. As I have said many times, thoughts (consciousness) are really things, creative particles that are constantly affecting the quantum field. When one is mindful of their own thoughts and has a defined purpose, the power of those thoughts is amazing.

Posture #3 - Earthship Maintenance:

Your body, your Earthship, is essential to your physical experience and if you take care of it, it will take care of you. A good diet and exercise plan are key to maintaining your body in good form. In the beginning, man had no choice but to eat real foods so eating natural was easy, there were no processed foods, no herbicides, pesticides, or chemical fertilizers and certainly no GMOs. Fortunately for most, today, if you shop smart, you can avoid most of the unnatural offerings, the ones that your body may recognize as a foreign invader.

You see, if anything you consume initiates your body's defense mechanisms, it uses up energy and resources while, at the same time, creating harmful substances. Real food, food that is itself healthy, speaks the language of your body, adds energy and adds to your resources.

Exercise is a bit simpler in that there are so many ways to stay fit. Simply focus on the three main areas of cardio, resistance and flexibility.

Cardio is just about getting moving enough to push your heart and lungs beyond their resting state. The more you push them the better they will perform for you. Only you know the level you require for the lifestyle you want to lead. And if you are not sure, check with a healthcare professional.

Resistance training is basically using weight or some other form of resistance against a movement of your body to grow your muscles and improve your endurance. Like the level of your cardio determining your heart health and lung capacity, the more the resistance the more your muscles will grow. Don't be one of the misinformed and spend endless hours with cardio and leave out the resistance exercise. Muscle development increases your metabolism so you burn more calories even in your sleep, making it easier to maintain a healthy weight. Building muscle also makes your bones stronger, your joints more sound, promotes youthful skin and you just plain look and feel better.

Form and balance are important not only for symmetrical development but also for protecting your body from injury. Be mindful of how you're moving and holding your body, not only when exercising but also throughout the day. Simply standing or sitting unevenly or unnecessarily tensing muscles, if repeated, can be an issue even for a healthy body.

Keep in mind that the genetics you were born with are just your body's original recipe, so be like a great chef and know that you can change the original and create the body you desire.

A fit and healthy body is fertile ground for applying your desires and beliefs. The forces that make positive creation and advanced evolution possible are being given the best possible message by a body for which there has been proper care.

Of course, the masses believe we should age in a certain way, but remember they are the same ones who are going through life with no real purpose but to get by. So if what you desire is a long, healthy life, then take good care of yourself and believe it is yours.

Posture #4 - Focus:

You will benefit by knowing what's going on in your head at all times! Most people have about 60,000 thoughts each and every day and 95% of them are the same thought. The worst part is 60% of those thoughts are negative and most are mindless, which means you aren't even aware you're thinking them. **So, essentially, at least 60% of the time you are programing yourself with stuff you probably don't want.** Instead of really seeing the world, you're unwittingly making your world less than it could be.

As I mentioned in Posture #2, focused belief is 10 times stronger—so why not make what's going on in your head work for you by being aware of what it is? When you think "purposely", those thoughts become productive tools of positive creation, which can take you to higher and higher levels.

With more focused thoughts you'll be able to slow down the chatter and pay more attention to what really matters, not only inside but outside as well. The world around you will seem to expand and instead of it being a passing blur, it will be an amazing display of wonder.

In a focused state you have an opportunity to feel better, be more productive, be a better listener and have a much happier life.

Synergy: With a focus on getting your thoughts under control, you get a huge boost for achieving what you desire in life and changing your beliefs. You eventually stop wasting time and energy creating things you don't want. **Your life's potential is huge, so why not make the best of it?**

If you have enjoyed this book and if you believe it was of some benefit, please pass it on to all your contacts. My goal is to improve as may lives as possible in as many ways as I can.

Reviews also help to spread the word and, again, if you like the book, I hope you will have the time to leave me a review as well.

If you feel a need to reach me please do at
crazyrichhealth@gmail.com

I would love to help!

Resources

I'm including these suggestions to get you started being proactive in finding answers for yourself. Answers to some of the questions you might have about your goal of being as healthy and happy as you can be. None of these sites are mine personally and are just examples.

And you can also reach me at crazyrichhealth@gmail.com if you have questions.

theheartysoul.com

This is a very comprehensive holistic health site. A good place to get more food and lifestyle ideas. Evidence and research based with contributors from in broad range of health modalities.

greenmedinfo.com

According to their site: they are "the world's most widely referenced, evidence-based, natural health resource with over 10,000 health topics and 50,000 peer reviewed abstracts."

Very alternative so you will need to be open to considering what is appropriate for you, but the research documents are there for your perusal.

livestrong.com

A good site for healthy promotion of a broad range of topics from good food tips to exercise advice. A bit more social than the previous sites but lots of good information. Like using avocado in place of butter in recipes or how to make a healthy alternative to ranch dressing that actually has only ingredients you can pronounce the name of.

Shaklee.com

Shaklee is a member oriented multilevel marketing company but you don't have to start a business to use their products. This is where I get my vitamin supplements because they have been proving themselves and their products since 1956. I am sure there are other companies who provide good supplements but I have been happy here for over 30 years at this point. Go to the About Us page for information on quality and effectiveness with references to the clinical research and testing that supports what they sell.

You can purchase at retail or pay a one-time fee of $19.99 and get a 15% discount. That can be done on the site or I'll be happy to guide you if you want to reach out to me at crazyrichhealth@gmail.com